A Collection of Proved Recipes for Common Diseases

常见病中医验方(秘方+偏方) 大全

Notes: the proved recipes listed herein are collected from the ancient Chinese medical works. Most of the ingredients of Traditional Chinese Medicine are common food ingredients, dried foods and coarse cereals, common plant leaves and stems and medical herbs, the preparation methods of these recipes are easy and simple, the proved recipes of TCM produce no side effect and are called biotherapy or naturopathy or green treatment.

Each proved recipe specifies the ingredients needed, preparation method, dosage, tips and warnings.

Unless otherwise specified, one recipe for one disease.

Table of Contents

1. Losing Weight
2. Fast Beauty
3. Removing Acne (2 Recipes)
4. Removing Black Nevus on the Face
5. Turing Premature Graying into Black Hair

(2 Recipes)
6. Hair Loss (Specific)
7. Not Drunk after Heavy Drinking
8. Discontinuing the Habit of Smoking and Drinking
9. Magic Therapy for Improving Intelligence Quotient
10. Beriberi   (5 Recipes)
11. Immediate and Radical Removal of Toothache   (9 Recipes)
12. Diarrhea Therapy (Acute Diarrhea & bowel disturbance Diarrhea)
13. Cold   (3 Recipes)
14. Cough
15. Hypertension   (9 Recipes)
16. Hypotension
17. Blood Lipid Thick   (3 Recipes)
18. Removing Freckles on the Face
19. Foot Sweat and Foot Odour
20. Neurasthenia
21. Stomatitis
22. Mouth Rote
23. Pharyngitis
24. Otitis Media
25. Tinnitus and Deafness
26. Migraine   (2 Recipes)
27. Trigeminal Autonomic Cephalalgias
28. Dizziness Headache
29. Hemorrhoids
30. Pruritus Vulvae and Rectal Itch
31. Epistaxis   (2 Recipes)
32. Rhinitis   (3 Recipes)

33. Glaucoma   (2 Recipes)
34. Eye Tears and Fungal Keratitis
35. Split Hand and Foot Malformation
36. Tache Noire
37. Periarthritis of Shoulder
38. Cholecystitis (including chronic cholecystitis) (3 Recipes)
39. Gastroenteritis
40. Rheumatoid Arthritis (2 Recipes)
41. Bronchitis   (3 Recipes)
42. Kidney Stone, urethral calculi, Gallstone   (4 Recipes)
43. Gastropathy (4 Recipes)
44. Bloating and Stomach Fullness
45. Numb limbs and sciatica
46. Ringworm of the Nails   (2 Recipes)
47. Magic Therapy for Warming Body in Cold Weather
48. Removing Red and Swollen Gums
49. Prostatitis   (2 Recipes)
50. Non-Acclimatization
51. Oral Ulcer   (2 Recipes)
52. Stomach Acid Reflux
53. Sprain
54. Senile Plaque
55. Removing Helosis
56. Cardia-Cerebrovascular Disease
57. Insomnia (Including hypertensive insomnia) (3 Recipes)
58. Oligophrenia Mutism
59. Tinnitus
60. Frequent Micturition (2 Recipes)

61. Dysentery
62. Varicosity (Applicable to the combined superficial phlebitis)
63. Psoriasis (3 Recipes)
64. Wart
65. Mildly Scalded
66. Pruritus
67. Vertigo
68. Asthma (2 Recipes)
69. Hypertensive Megrim
70. Hand and Foot Injuries (Blood Disorder)
71. Constipation (2 Recipes)
72. Cerebral Thrombosis, Cerebral Infarction
73. Spur
74. Nasosinusitis
75. Premature Beat
76. Prostatic Hyperplasia
77. Foot Stomium
78. Traumatic Injury
79. Duodenal Ulcer (2 Recipes)
80. Urinary Incontinence
81. Hyperostosis (2 Recipes)
82. Decreasing Blood Pressure (3 Recipes)
83. Peritus Ani
84. Throat Inflammation, sore red swollen throat caused by Cold and Fever
85. Pruritus
86. Anemia
87. Ulcerative Colitis
88. Gastroptosis
89. Red and White Dysentery
90. Diabetes

91. Esophagitis, Throat Dumb
92. Pneumonia
93. Rheumatism
94. Low Back Pain
95. Dizziness, Headache
96. Epigastric Pain
97. Stomachache
98. Hepatitis
99. Female Infertility
100. Amenorrhoea
101. Irregular Menstruation
102. Menstrual Pain
103. Leucorrhea
104. Magic Method for Promoting Lactation
105. Persistent Menstruation
106. Gastrorrhagia
107. Impotence
108. Baby Night Cry
109. Verminal Invasion Ear
110. Foot Crack
111. Toe Corns and wart
112. Burn Injury (Scald)
113. Venomous Snake Bite
114. Enuresis, Trickling
115. Enterobiasis
116. Edema
117. Urinary Stoppage
118. Stool Indigestion
119. Body Itch
120. Bed-Wetting
121. Otitis
122. Common Eye Diseases

123. Sore on the Back
124. Dreaminess after Sleeping
125. Fishbone Stuck in Throat
126. Paralysis
127. Acne
128. Deviation of Mouth and Eye
129. Hernia
130. Vitiligo
131. Lichen Planus
132. Carsickness
133. Gas Poisoning
134. Stop Nosebleed
135. Stop Bleeding Knife Wound
136. Skin Diseases of the Scrota
137. Food Poisoning
138. Obesity
139. Night Blindness
140. Measle Prevention
141. Flat Wart
142. Indigestion
143. Body Odor
144. Dysentery
145. Hypochromic Anemia, Dizziness Insomnia
146. Dry throat and mouth, feverishness in palms and soles
147. Ozostomia

A Collection of Proved Recipes for Common Diseases

常见病中医验方(秘方+偏方)大全

1. 变瘦
1. Losing Weight

配方：红豆100克，绿豆100克，山楂30克，大枣10枚。
Ingredients: 100g red beans, 100g green bean, 30g hawthorn, 10 jujubes.

做法：将所有材料共放在锅中，加1000毫升冷水，煎到豆烂即可。
Method: Put all the ingredients into a pot, then add 1000ml cold water, cook the ingredients till the beans become pulpy.

温馨提示：红豆和绿豆煮之前最好用冷水泡一个小时，会比较容易煮烂的。
Tips: Soak the red bean and green bean in cold water for one hour before cooking, so that the red bean and green bean will be more easy to become pulpy in cooking.

食用方法：做好后，分两等份，一份趁热时，连汤带豆和山楂，枣一起吃下。另外一份就用保鲜膜包好放冰箱中冷藏，吃之前热一下。
Dosage: After the work is done, divide the food of into two equal units, eat one unit while it is hot, store another unit in

refrigerator for eating next time. Heat it again before eating.

原理：红豆，绿豆都是排毒圣品，并且有高纤维低脂肪的特点。山楂健脾开胃，消食减脂。红枣调和胃气补血润燥。此方共用，有助各种单品的功效最大限度的发挥。

Theory: Red bean and green bean have good function of detoxifying and featured with high fiber and low fat. Hawthorn is appetizer that can reduce fat. The red jujube can regulate stomach and enrich the blood. This recipe mixes these ingredients together and maximizes their functions.

为取得更好的减肥效果，期间应严格遵守以下生活规律：

In order to achieve better weight loss effect, the following pattern of life should be observed during the use of the recipe:

- 每天起床后首先喝一杯蜜醋水，这是减肥汤。作法：在 250 毫升的温开水中加入一汤匙蜂蜜和 1/4 汤匙的醋(最好是白醋)，搅拌均匀后作为早餐喝下。
- Drink a cup of honey vinegar after getting up every morning, it is a weight-losing soup. Method: add one spoon of honey and 1/4 spoon vinegar (white vinegar preferred), stir it to an even state, and drink it as breakfast.
- 中餐吃上述减肥粥，上下午时间光不吃任何零食。
- Eat the above weight-losing porridge as the lunch, do not eat any snacks during the day
- 晚餐也只吃上述减肥粥，在 7 点之前吃完，吃完后睡觉前绝不吃任何食物。

- Eat the same porridge as supper before seven o'clock in the evening, and do not any food before going to bed.

2. 快速美容
2. Fast Beauty

鸡蛋三个，用酒泡，密封4至7天，每天以蛋清涂面，七天面如白雪。
Ingredients: 3 eggs, soak the eggs in wine for 4 to 7 days, coat the face with egg white each day. Seven days later, the face will look like white snow.

3. 治青春痘
3. Removing Acne

(1) 用蒲公英2两，熬水喝，一天一付，半月治愈。
(1) 60g dandelion, cook it in hot water and drink it once a day, the acne will be removed half a month later.
(2) 白芷30克、盐10克。每天用上药泡水2小时外用，搽患处。
(2) 30g Rhizoma Bletillae. 30g salt, soak them in the water for two hours, apply the drug on the area of acne.

4. 脸上黑痣点去掉法
4. Removing Black Nevus on the Face

生石灰、白碱各一半，用酒精调成糊状，点在黑痣上半天即掉。

Put equal portion of quicklime and dietary alkali into the alcohol, stir them till the ingredients become pasty, apply the drug on the black nevus on the face, the black nevus will be removed half a day later.

5. 少白头变黑发
5. Turing Premature Graying into Black Hair

(1) 柏壳装枕头，枕半年自黑。
(1) Fill the pillow with shell of cypress seeds, sleep on such pillow each night, the grey hair will turn into black half a year later.
(2) 何首乌三两，黑芝麻三两加红糖水煮沸分三次吃完。连吃半月后，白发逐渐变黑。
(2) Take 90g polygonum multiflorum, 90g black sesame, put them into the brown sugar water, cook the water till it boils, eat up the drug in three times, the grey hair will become black half a month later.

6. 治头发脱落特效法
6. Hair Loss (Specific)

用桑叶熬水洗头，三日即愈。
Soak the mulberry leaf into water, wash the head with the water, the effect will come three days later.

7. 千杯不醉法
7. Not Drunk after Heavy Drinking

樟木、葛根各半两泡茶喝，饮酒前喝下防醉，醉后喝下解酒。

15g camphor wood, 15g Radix Puerariae, put them into the tea water, cook it till the water boils. Drink the tea water before drinking wine for anti-intoxication, and drink it after getting drunk for de-alcoholic.

8. 戒烟、戒酒法
8. Discontinuing the Habit of Smoking and Drinking

用南瓜秧焙干研面冲水当茶喝，至不想吸为止（戒烟）。

Bake pumpkin sprouts to dried, smash the dried sprouts into the powder, put the power into water, cook the tea water till it boils, drink the water as tea till the habit of smoking disappears.

马在出汗时，刮下25克马汗，用500克开水搅拌均喝下（戒酒）。

When a horse sweats, scrap 25g horse sweat, put the horse sweat into 500g boiled water, stir the boiled water evenly, drink the water, the habit of drinking will be removed gradually.

9. 开智商妙方
9. Magic Therapy for Improving Intelligence Quotient

荷花梗晒干为沫，同何首乌，滚水冲服当茶，久则聪明，虽至愚者亦心灵生慧也。
Dry the lotus stalk, smash it into powder, then put the powder and polygonum multiflorum into boiling water, drink the water as tea for a long time, the intelligence quotient will be improved gradually.

10. 治脚气
10. Beriberi

(1) 韭菜一斤，煮水十分钟泡脚，每日一次，每次20分钟，三天除根。
(1) 500g fragrant-flowered garlic, cook it in water for 10 minutes, then soak the foot into the water for 20 minutes, do it once every day, the Beriberi will be removed three days later.

(2) 柳树叶50克，鲜柳树叶用刀剁碎，早上放在袜子里，每天放一次，当天见效，四天可治愈。
(2) 50g willow leaves, mince the leaves into pieces, put the pieces into the sock, do it once a day, the Beriberi will be removed four days later.

(3) 脚趾缝溃烂时，摘几片最嫩的柳叶，将其搓成小丸状，夹在脚趾缝溃烂处，晚上夹入后再穿上袜子，以防滑掉，第二天就可见效，3天脚气即可治愈。脚气大面积发病时，可将嫩柳叶一把加水煎熬，然后用煎熬的温水洗脚，也可以起到立竿见影的效果，脚气3~5天即可痊愈。
(3) When the bare toes fester, pick several most tender willow leaves, rub them into small balls, put them onto the toes festering area, wear sock at night to prevent falling off,

do it for three days, Beriberi will be removed. When the Beriberi spreads extensively, pick a bundle of tender willow leaves into water, then cook the water till the water boils, then wash the foot with the warm boiled water, do it once a day, the Beriberi will be removed 3-5 days later.

(4) 用吸过的烟头，夹在脚趾头当中，三日痊愈。
(4) Clamp the smoked cigarette among the toes, the Beriberi will be removed three days later.

(5) 每天睡觉前用温水洗脚后,用棉签蘸适量风油精涂于患处,一般连续使用5天,就能基本达到止痛、止痒的作用。如果伴有水疱，应先用针将水疱挑破，再用风油精。

(5) After washing foot before going to bed, dip cotton swab into essential balm, then wipe the Beriberi area, repeat it for consecutive five days, the pain and itch will be removed. If there is blister, break it, then wipe the Beriberi with cotton swab dipped with essential balm.

11. 立治和根治牙疼
11. Immediate and Radical Removal of Toothache

(1) 红霉素片3粒 + 维生素B1（4粒）+ 维生素B2（2粒）开水送服，一天两次，半小时止痛。
(1) 3 pieces of Erythromycin Tablets + 4 pieces of Vitamin B1 + 2 pieces of Vitamin B2, take them together with boiled water, do it twice a day, the toothache will be removed half an hour later.

(2) 取大蒜适量捣烂，温热后敷在痛点上可以缓解牙髓炎、牙周炎以及牙痛等症状。
(2) Take some garlic and mash it into pulp, warm it, then apply it on the pain spot, the pulpitis, Periodontitis and toothache can be alleviated.

(3) 把味精与温开水按 1：50 的比例化开后，口含味精溶液一会儿再吐掉。这样连续几次，坚持两天后牙痛就会消失。
(3) Mix aginomoto with warm water at the ratio of 1:50, then hold the aginomoto solution in mouth for a moment, then spit out the solution, repeat it for several times, do it for two days, the toothache will disappear.

(4) 牙痛的时候可以切一片小生姜咬在痛处，必要的时候可以重复使用。
(4) Cut a small ginger, bit the ginger at the pain point, and repeat it when necessary.

(5) 取白酒 100 克放在杯中，再加食盐 10 克，搅拌，等食盐溶化后烧开。含上一口在疼痛的地方（不要咽下去），牙痛会立即止住。
(5) Put 100g white spirit into the cup, add 10g salt the white spirit, stir the white spirit. After the salt dissolves, cook the solution to boiled, hold appropriate amount of the solution in mouth for a moment (do not swallow the solution down), the toothache will be removed right away.

(6) 叩——固齿。每日早晚各一次，每次 3~5 分钟。叩时用力发出响声。
(6) Knock ----- strengthening teeth. Do it once for 3-5 minutes in the morning and evening, make sound when

knocking.

(7) 咬——防、治牙痛。大小便时尤为重要，最好平时经常咬（即所谓咬紧牙关），也有好处。
(7) Grit ----- Preventing and controlling toothache. It is particularly important to grit at the time of defecation, gritting at ordinary times is recommended (so called "clench one's teeth").

(8) 白酒一两，松香 15 克，泡 2 小时后用棉花沾酒放在牙疼处，咬紧。5 分钟不疼，
(8) Take 30g white spirit, 15g rosins, soak the rosins into white spirit for 2 hours, then use the cotton swab to dip the solution on the pain point, clench the teeth, the toothache will disappear five minutes later.

(9) 蚂蜂窝．红糖各 1 两，兑两碗水，煎剩下一碗半时让患者喝下，三十年不疼。
(9) take 30g hornet cellular, 30g brown sugar, mix them in the water of two bowls, cook the water to boiling till the water decreases to the volume of one and half of bowls of water, drink the cooled water, the toothache will be removed permanently.

12. 治腹泻 (包括急性腹泻&肠紊乱腹泻)
12. Diarrhea Therapy (Acute Diarrhea & bowel disturbance Diarrhea)

- 治急性腹泻
- **Acute Diarrhea**

一般的用保济丸即可，如果较严重，用氟哌酸搞定。

Use health pill to cure ordinary Acute Diarrhea, if the condition is severe, use norfloxacin to stop Acute Diarrhea.

- 治肠紊乱腹泻
- Bowel Disturbance Diarrhea

把一个苹果（带皮）洗净后，切成八、九块，放一大碗水，用小火煮，等苹果煮烂，连果带汤吃下，每天早晚各吃一次，十来天后大便成形，一个月后恢复如初。

Cut a washed apple (with skin) into eight and nine pieces, put these pieces into a big bowl of water, cook the water till the pieces become tender. Drink such apple soup once in the morning and evening respectively, the defecate will form ten days later and will resume normal one month later.

13. 治感冒

13. Cold

(1) 香菜一把，葱白连须 5 根，生姜 10 片，水煎，加红糖一两，趁热服，一天两次，一天治愈。

(1) A bundle of coriander, 5 pieces of fistular onion stalk with roots, 10 pieces of ginger, cook them in water till boiled, add 30g brown sugar to the boiled water, cool the water for a moment, then eat the soup twice a day, the cold will be removed in a day.

(2) 将新鲜白菜根一个洗净，加红糖 30 克和老姜五片，水煎服。每日一剂一服，连服三日见效。

(2) Clean the fresh cabbage roots, 30g brown sugar and 5 pieces of old ginger, cook them in the water till boiled, take one dosage a day, repeat it for consecutive three days.

(3) 生姜 10 片，白萝卜 10 片，加红糖煎服，服后发汗。一次即愈。

(3) 10 pieces of ginger, 10 pieces of white turnip, some brown sugars, cook them in water till boiled, take the dosage, the body will sweat, the cold will be removed.

14. 治咳嗽
14. Cough

(1) 白菜根两棵洗净，冰糖 30 克，共用水煮，喝汤。注意：针对咳嗽、痰多病症。

(1) Clean two cabbage roots, 30g rock candy, cook them in water, drink the soup, this recipe is right for cough with phlegm.

15. 治高血压
15. Hypertension

(1）香蕉皮 30 克，晒干水煎喝，每日 3 次，一个月见效。

(1) 30 banana skin, dry it, cook it in water till boiled, drink the soup three times a day, the effect will come one month later.

(2）用中药罗布麻，开水冲喝，每日 15 克，半月见效。

(2) Cook the Apocynum venetum in water till boiled, the effect will come half a month later.

(3) 用蜂蜜 100 克，黑芝麻 75 克，先将黑芝麻蒸熟捣如泥，放蜂蜜搅拌，用温开水冲化，每日分 2 次服用。
每日早晚各一杯纯蜂蜜水，会使血压趋于正常。

(3) 100g honey, 75g black sesame, steam the black sesame to squashy, then mash the black sesame to the mud like, add the honey to the sesame mud, stir it, pour the hot boiled water to the mixed honey and sesame, drink the soup twice a day.

(4) 银杏叶每日 15 克，用开水冲喝下，半月见效。
(4) Take 15g gingko leaf each day, put the gingko leaf into boiling water, drink the water, the effect will come half a month later.

(5) 花生半碗（大碗，带红衣）加上好醋慢一碗．泡上 7 天，每天早晚各吃１０粒．等血压降下来后可改为几天服用一次．巩固疗效．主治：清热活血，用治高血压，对保护血管壁，阻止血栓形成有较好的作用（高血压）。
(5) A big bowl of peanut (with red skin), a bow of good vinegar, soak the peanut in vinegar for 7 days, eat 10 such soaked peanuts every morning and evening. After the blood pressure decreases, eat the peanuts once every several days to consolidate the effect. The function of this therapy is to clear heat and activate blood, this therapy has good effect in protecting vessel wall and blocking the formation of thrombus.

(6) 白胡椒 7 粒，南杏仁 4 粒，糯米 7 粒，桃仁 2 两，枝子 1 两。
(6) Ingredients: 7 white peppers, 4 southern apricot kernels, 7 pieces of glutinous rice, 60g peach seeds, 30g twigs.

方法：将上列五物研成粉末，用鸡蛋的蛋白混合后，捏成饼状。晚上睡前贴在脚底心上。男左女右，用纱布包好。第二天早晨起床后除去。（一副只能用一次）。如脚上发现有青色，乃正常现象。轻者三服，重者五服，连续使用，不可隔天。

注意：此方忌口服。次方根除高血压。

Method: Smash the above ingredients into powder, then mix with egg white, crush them a pie like, past the pie on arch of the foot (left for male and right for female), wrap the foot with gauze before going to bed, remove the gauze after getting up early next morning. If there is cyan, it is the normal symptom. Do the same for consecutive three to five times.

Warning: this dosage shall not be taken orally.

(7) 花生全草（整棵草）一次 50 克，切段煎水．干品一次 50 克，鲜品一次 150 克．一它一剂．血压正后可改为不定期服用．巩固疗效。

主治：清热凉血，有降血压，降胆固醇作用，对治疗高血压有较理想的功效。

(7) Take 50g dried peanut herb (whole), or 150g fresh peanut herb, cut the herb into several sections, cook the sections in water till boiled, drink the dosage once a day. After the blood pressure returns to normal, take the dosage from time to time to consolidate the effect.

The therapy can clear the heat, cool the blood and lower cholesterol and has good effect.

8）用玉米穗上的须熬水当茶喝，半月即愈。

(8) Take some stigma maydis, cook them in water till boiled, drink the water as tea, the effect will come half a month later.

(9) 用蜂蜜 100 克,黑芝麻 75 克,先将黑芝麻蒸熟捣如泥,放蜂蜜搅拌,用温开水冲化,每日分 2 次服用。每日早晚各一杯纯蜂蜜水,会使血压趋于正常。

(9) 100g honey, 75g black sesame, steam the black sesame, then smash it into powder like, then mix honey with the black sesame and pour warm boiled water to the mixed honey and black sesame. Take the dosage twice a day, drink a cup of pure honey water, the blood pressure will return to normal.

16. 治低血压
16. Hypotension

甘草 20 克,桂枝,肉桂各 40 克,将以上药物混合后当茶冲泡服用一周。

20g radix glycyrrhizae, 40g cassia twig, 40g cinnamon, mix these ingredients, and put them into boiling water, then drink the water as tea for one week.

17. 治血脂稠
17. Blood Lipid Thick

(1) 枸杞子 10 克,何首乌,草决明,山楂各 15 克,丹参 20 克,水煎服,每日两次,四个疗程治愈,(七天为一个疗程)。

(1) 10g fructus lycii, 15g polygonum multiflorum, 15g Cassia occidentalis, 15g hawthorn, 20g salviae miltiorrhizae, cook these ingredients in water till boiled, then drink the dosage twice a day, lasting four treatment

courses (one treatment course is 7 days).

(2) 山楂，银杏叶， 绞股蓝各 15 克，泡茶喝。连服四疗程（半月为一个疗程）
(2) 15g hawthorn, 15g ginkgo leaf, 15g gynostemma pentaphyllum, cook them in water till boiled, drink the dosage as tea, lasting four treatment courses (one treatment course is 15 days)

(3) 花生米 1 两，陈醋半斤，泡七天后服用，每日 3 次，每次吃 2 个。
(3) take 30g peanuts, 250g mature vinegar, soak the peanuts in mature vinegar for seven days, then eat two peanuts once, do it three times a day.

18. 治脸上黑星（雀斑）
18. Removing Freckles on the Face

元荽（又名香菜），煎汤，天天洗 （一天三次为佳），数日去除。
Take some coriander, cook them in water till boiled, then use the soup to wash the freckles on the face every day, do it three times a day, the freckles will be removed in a few days later.

19. 治脚汗，脚臭
19. Foot Sweat and Foot Odour

白萝卜煮水，每晚熏洗双脚 30 分钟，连洗半月治愈。
Cook the white radish in water till boiled, use the water to

wash the foot every evening, the foot sweat and foot odour will be removed half a month later.

20. 治神经衰弱
20. Neurasthenia

浮小麦50克，干草24克，大枣20克，酸枣仁30克，混合。水煎服，每天一次，半月治愈。
50g light wheat, 24g radix glycyrrhizae, 20g jujube, 30g semen ziziphi spinosae, mix these ingredients together, then cook them in water till boiled, take the dosage once a day, the effect will come half a month later.

21. 治口腔炎
21. Stomatitis

西瓜皮晒干，烽炒焦，加冰片少许研末，用蜂蜜调和涂于患处，特效。
Dry the watermeion peel, cook the honey to caramel colour, mix the two with a little borneol, grind the mixed ingredients into powder, add honey to the powder and stir, apply the dosage to the affected part, the dosage is very effective.

22. 治烂嘴
22. Mouth Rote

用浓茶叶水，加少许食盐，然后用来漱口，一天三至五次，三日治愈。

Add a little salt to strong tea water, rinse the mouth with such tea water three to five times a day, the disease will be cured three days later.

23. 治咽炎
23. Pharyngitis

取芦荟叶二至三片（大的二片或小的三片），用清水洗净，切成小段，放入锅内。加水（一至二碗）和冰糖适量（以甜为度）共煮沸后十分钟，用纱布过滤，去渣，取其液当开水喝，两天见效，五至七天痊愈。

Take two to three pieces of aloe barbadensis leaf, wash them, then cut them into small sections, and put them into pot. Add water (one to two bowls) and some rock candy to the pot, cook the ingredients till the water boils, and ten minutes later, use the gauze to filter the water, drink the filtered liquid as boiled water, the disease will be cured within five to seven days.

24. 治中耳炎
24. Otitis Media

韭菜根一两捣烂，挤出水份，加入少许冰片，滴耳，特效。

Take 30g leek root, mash it into pulp, squeeze the water in it, add a little borneol to the water, drop the water on the ear, the dosage is very effective.

25. 治耳鸣耳聋

25. Tinnitus and Deafness

雄乌鸡一只，甜酒四斤，煮熟后趁热吃，连吃五只，特效。

One male blackone chicken, 2kg sweet wine, cook the chicken in sweet wine thoroughly, eat five such chickens continuously, this dosage is very effective.

26. 治偏头疼
26. Migraine

(1) 生萝卜汁适量，用法：仰卧注入鼻中，左痛注右，右痛注左，神效，如加冰片少许更妙。

(1) Take some raw radish juice. Method: lie on back, pour the raw radish juice into nose. If the headache is on left, pour the raw radish juice on right nostril, and vice versa, the effect is very good, It will be better if a little borneol is added.

(2) 偏头痛症通常是由于大脑供氧过量引起的，当偏头痛症刚发作时，拿一个圆锥形的小纸袋或小塑料袋（最好不透孔），将袋子开口的一头捂住鼻子和嘴，用力向袋内呼气，以减少大脑的氧气，反复数次后，偏头痛症就会缓解，以致最后消失。

(2) Migraine is usually caused by oversupply of oxygen to brain. When migraine occurs, take a conical paper bag or plastic bag, cover it on the nose and mouth, blow into the bag with force to reduce the oxygen of the brain. Repeat the action for several times, Migraine will be alleviated and disappear in the end.

27. 治神经头痛
27. Trigeminal Autonomic Cephalalgias

白芷4克，冰片2克，细辛2克，研成粉卷入纸筒放药粉燃着，用鼻吸入烟气.
4g Angelica dahurica, 2g borneol, 2g asarum, grind these ingredients into powder, put the powder into paper tube, burn the paper tube, inhale the smoke into nose.

28. 治头晕头痛
28. Dizziness Headache

黄芪. 天麻各一两，炖黄母鸡一只吃下，连吃三只治愈。
Take 30g astragalus, 30g gastrodin, stew a yellow hen with 50g astragalus and 50g gastrodin.

29. 治痔疮
29. Hemorrhoids

皮硝一两，槐米半斤。熬水熏洗，洗患处，每日两次，七天治愈。治外痔特效。
Take 30g Mirabilite, 250g pagodatree flower bud, boil the gradients in water, wash the affected part with the water, the Hemorrhoids will be cured seven days later.

30. 治阴痒肛痒
30. Pruritus Vulvae and Rectal Itch

醋 500 克，盐 5 克加热洗，一天三次。
500g vinegar, 5g salt, mix and heat them, wash the affected part three times a day.

31. 治鼻出血
31. Epistaxis

(1) 左鼻出血从右耳吹气，右鼻出血从左耳吹气，可立即止血。
(1) Blow the air into right ear if left nostril bleeds, vice versa, the bleeding can be stopped immediately.

(2) 用头发烧成灰吹入鼻孔立止（男用母发，女用父发）可根除。
(2) Burn the hair into ash, blow the ash into nostril (the mother's hair is used for male patient, and father's hair is used for female patient)

32. 治鼻炎
32. Rhinitis

(1) 苍耳子 30 克，轻轻捣烂放入小勺内，加香油 50 克火煎，将苍耳子碎渣捞出，用油滴鼻子，一天 3 至 5 次。

(1) 30g siberian cocklour fruit, mash it into small pieces, put the pieces into spoon, add 50g sesame oil to the pieces, then fry the pieces with fire, extract siberian cocklour fruit, drop the sesame oil into the noise, do it three to five times a day.

(2) 用砖和瓦上的青醭，焙干研碎成粉，撒入鼻孔，每天三次，三日除根。
(2) Take some moss growing on the bricks and tiles, bake them to dried, then mash them into powder, throw the powder into nostril, do it three times a day, the Rhinitis will be eradicated three days later.

(3) 每天吃饭时，随同饭菜同吃一些生大葱。在吃的过程中，口中多嚼一会儿，让大葱的辣味从鼻孔中通过，这样效果会更好。
(3) Eat some welsh onion with daily meal, chew the welsh onion more time to make the peppery taste pass through the nostril, the effect will be better.

33. 治青光眼
33. Glaucoma

(1) 向日葵盘（去籽）3朵，斩碎水煎一半内服另一半熏洗眼部半月治愈。
(1) Take 3 sunflower heads (remove the seeds), cut them into pieces, boil the pieces in water. Take half the dosage orally, the another half is used to fumigate the eyes, the Glaucoma will be cured half a month later.

(2) 急性青光眼病人，可服蜂蜜80毫升，一日分三次服完；慢性青光眼、眼压持续偏高者，服蜂蜜50毫升，一日分3次服完，几天后可使症状缓解。因蜂蜜是一种高渗剂，服后能使血液渗透压升高，以吸收眼内水分，降低眼压。
(2) In the case of acute Glaucoma, eat 80ml honey up in

three times a day; in the case of chronic glaucoma and continuous high intraocular pressure, eat 50ml honey up in three times a day. As honey is a high osmotic agent, it can promote the rise of blood osmotic pressure to absorb the water in the eye and lower intraocular pressure.

34. 治眼流泪，角膜炎
34. Eye Tears and Fungal Keratitis

鱼苦胆点眼，一天三次，半月治愈。
Drop fish gall in eyes, do it three times a day, the effect will come half a month later.

35. 治手足裂
35. Split Hand and Foot Malformation

五倍子适量研末，用牛骨髓或矾士林调涂抹缝中，五日治愈。
Take some gallnut, grind them into powder, mix bovine bone marrow or vaseline with the powder, apply the mixed powder in the cracks, the effect will come five days later.

36. 治黑斑
36. Tache Noire

当归半斤，煮水一碗，用此水抹患处，半月见效。
250g angelica sinensis, boil it in the water of a bowl, apply the water on the affected part, the effect will come half a month.

37. 治肩关节周炎
37. Periarthritis of Shoulder

生姜一两，芋头二两，去皮捣烂如泥，用布袋装好贴患处，一天两次，四个疗程治愈（七天为一个疗程）。
30g ginger, 60g taro, peel off the skin of the ingredients, mix and smash them into the mud like, put the dosage into cloth bag, past the dosage on the affected part, do it twice a day, four treatment courses are needed (one treatment course is seven days)

38. 治胆囊炎 (包括慢性胆囊炎)
38. Cholecystitis (including chronic cholecystitis)

(1) 玉米须 30 克，蒲公英，茵陈各 15 克。水煎服，每日三次，一个月治愈。
(1) 30g corn stigma, 15g dandelion, 15g capillary Artemisia, mix these ingredients and boil them in water, drink the dosage soup three times a day, the effect will come one month later.

(2) 慢性胆囊炎：柳树叶可入药，有消炎、解毒、利尿的功效。春天柳树发芽后采集，制成茶叶，天天饮用，能治愈。
(2) chronic cholecystitis: willow leaves are medical herb and have the functions of anti-inflammation, detoxification and diuresis. Collect the willow leaves in spring, make them into tea leaves, drink such tea water every day, chronic cholecystitis will be cured.

(3) 每天清早空腹吃一个苹果(连皮一起食用)，隔半小时后再进餐。一年 365 天，每天坚持。
(3) Eat an apple first after getting up every morning (not peel off the skin the apple), then have breakfast half an hour later, do it around the year.

39. 治肠胃炎
39. Gastroenteritis

木瓜 100 克，扁豆 100 克，兑水煮熟吃豆喝汤，一天两次，半月除根。
100g pawpaw, 100g hyacinth bean, boil them in water thoroughly, then eat the hyacinth bean and drink the soup, do it twice a day, Gastroenteritis will be eradicated half a month later.

40. 治类风湿性关节炎
40. Rheumatoid Arthritis

(1) 辣椒 2 两泡白酒 2 斤，泡七天后洗患处，一天三次，半月治愈。
(1) take 60g pepper, 1000g white spirit, soak the pepper in the white spirit for seven days, wash the affected part with the liquid, do it three times a day, the effect will come half a month.

(2) 用野线麻叶裹住关节，多用几层，3 日换一次，多换几次，关节部位逐渐好转。
(2) Wrap up the joint with Boehmeria gracilis, more layers

are preferred, change the Boehmeria gracilis once three days, do it several times, the joint will turn well gradually.

41. 治气管炎
41. Bronchitis

(1) 炒桃仁，白胡椒，枝子，乙醚各 25 克，碾成碎面，鸡蛋清调和，男左女右贴在脚心处，吃鸡蛋。每天一个，七天特效。
(1) 25g fried peach seed, 25g white pepper, 25g cape jasmine, 25g diethyl ether, grind these ingredients into chips, then mix with egg white, apply the mixed dosage in the arch of the foot, eat one egg a day, the effect will come seven days later.

(2) 每天早晨将一个新鲜鸡蛋打入碗中，搅均后备用。先将竹叶（中药店有售）洗净放在水中煮，煮沸后把竹叶捞出，然后将烧开的竹叶水冲入准备好的鸡蛋中，用碟子盖好，闷上一会儿即可，每天早晨空腹服用一次。蛋中不要放任何调料，尤其是盐。坚持服用 15~20 天，慢性支气管炎会有效果。
(2) Open one fresh egg every morning, put it into a bow and stir the egg evenly, put it aside. Wash the bamboo leaves and boil them in water till boiled, pour the boiled bamboo leaves water into the ready egg bowl, cover the bowl for a moment, then drink the egg soup with empty stomach, keep on doing so for 15-20 days, the effect will come. Warning: do not put any flavor, including salt, into the egg soup.

(3) 喝大豆腐水，连续喝多日;神奇般的根除。

(3) Drink soft beancurd water for consecutive days, the disease will be removed.

42. 治肾结石，尿道结石，胆结石
42. Kidney Stone, urethral calculi, Gallstone

(1) 鸡内金 10 克，焙干研末，白开水冲服，一天三次，一个月治愈。
(1) 10g chickens gizzard-membrane, dry it and grind it into the powder, put the powder into boiling water, then drink the water, do it three times a day, the disease will be cured one month later.

(2) 香油（芝麻油）500 克，核桃仁 500 克，冰糖 500 克，装盆，上锅蒸（冰糖化为止）。蒸好后分九份，每天服一份。
(2) 500g sesame oil, 500g walnut kernel, 500g rock candy, steam the ingredients in pot (till the rock candy melts), then divide the dosage into nine parts, take one part orally each day.

(3) 虎杖 60 克，茵陈 30 克，大黄 15 克。水煎服，每日二次。
(3) 60g polygonum cuspidatum, 30g Herba Artemisiae scopariae, 15g rhubarb, boil the ingredients in water till boiled, drink the soup twice a day.

(4) 核桃仁，冰糖各 20 克，香油 50 克，温开水冲服，每天一剂，一个月治愈。
(4) 20g walnut kernel, 20g rock candy, 50g sesame oil, put these ingredients into hot boiled water, take one dosage a

day, the disease will be cured one month later.

43. 治胃病
43. Gastropathy

(1) 配方：乌贼骨 150 克、制元胡 50 克、黄氏 50 克、鸡内金 150 克、制白术 50 克、猪苓 50 克、乌梅 50 克、大黄 5 克。
(1) Ingredients: 150g cuttlebone, 50g rhizoma corydalis, 50g Gum tragacanth, 150g chickens gizzard-membrane, 20g rhizoma atractylodis macrocephalae, 50g Polyporus umbellate, 50g fructus mume, 5g rhubarb.

此方通治：各类胃炎、溃疡、胀痛、消化不良、胃肠动力不足、肠炎等一切胃肠疾病。
买药时在药店加工成粉，如果胃寒或胃凉者加良姜 50 克。
This recipe is applicable to: gastritis, ulcer, distending pain, dyspepsia, Gastrointestinal motility disorder, enteritis and other gastrointestinal diseases. In case of stomach cold or cool, add some falangal as case may be (50g is the most).
Method: grind these ingredients into powder, boiled the powder in water till boiled and make it as dosage soup.

服法： 一天两到三次，饭前一小时或半小时各服一汤勺（6--10 克）。严重者可以每次加服云南白药一粒。重者一般 3 到 5 天见效，轻者一次见效．一般 1--2 副药可以根治。有效率 98%。无任何负作用。
Instructions: Take one spoon of the soup (6-10g) orally one or half an hour prior to meal, do it two or three times a day, the effect will be seen 3 to 5 days later. If the state is

not serious, the disease can be eradicated after taking 1~ 2 dosages of the drug and no side effect will produce.

注意：不要吃冷的，冻的，凉性的食物。不要饿过头，也不要吃饱，保持在七八分饱就好。不要吃完饭就躺下。一天空腹服药三次或四次，也可以在痛时或胀时服药．东西不要煮烂吃。

Warnings: do not eat cold, frozen and cool food, do not get too hungry and eat too much. Do not lie down after a meal, take the dosage three or four times a day with empty stomach or take the dosage at the time of stomachache or gastrectasia.

(2）配方：浮小麦 50 克(浮小麦，尖尖长长，有外羽，很轻．主治失眠)．甘草 10 克，灵芝 15 克，红枣 15 个，白术 10 克，党参 10 克，北芪 1 5 克，黄芪 10 克，淮山 20 克，丹参 10 克，田七 10 克。

(2) **Ingredients:** 50g light wheat, 10g liquorice, 15g ganoderma lucidum, 15 red jujubes, 10g Atractylodes, 10g codonopsis pilosula, 15g astragalus, 10g astraglus base, 20g Chinese yam, 10g root of red-rooted salvia, 10g pseudo-ginseng.

煎法：将药洗净，同煎．红枣要切两半．
Preparation Method: cut each red jujube into two halves, clean these ingredients, boil them together till the water boiled.

服法：一天一剂，7 天为一疗程．连服 3 — 4 疗程．药煎两次．饭后一小时服或空腹服。
Instructions: Boil the medicine twice, take one dosage a day one hour later after meal or with empty stomach, 3-4

treatment courses are required, one treatment course is 7 days.

(3) 配方：血灵脂 25 克，延胡素，香附佛手各 20 克，甘松 15 克，水煎服。一天一剂，半月治愈。
(3) **Ingredients:** 25g ganoderma lucidum, 20g rhizoma corydalis, 20g Rhizoma cyperi bergamot, 15g nardostachyos, boil the ingredients in water till boiled, take one dosage a day, the effect will come half a month later.

(4) 配方：人丹 12 包，香附子半斤，研面分 20 份，每日 3 次，每次 1 包，两剂即愈。
(4) **Ingredients**: 12 bags of rendan mini-pills, 250g cyperus rotundus, grind the ingredients into flour, and divide the flour into 20 equal units, take one unit each time, do the same three times a day, the effect will come after two treatment courses.

44. 治胃胀胃满
44. Bloating and Stomach Fullness

黑白丑焙干研末，白开水冲服，每天 3 次，每次 10 克，七日治愈。
Take 10g semen pharbitidis, dry semen pharbitidis, grind it into powder, then put the powder into boiling water, drink the soup three times a day, the disease will be cured seven days later.

45. 治四肢麻木，坐骨神经疼
45. Numb limbs and sciatica

生姜，大蒜各20克，切碎拌陈醋100克，加水一碗煎开熏洗患处。

Ingredients: 20g fresh ginger, 20g garlic, cut them into pieces, stir the pieces with 100g mature vinegar, then put them into pot, pour a bowl of water into the pot, boil the ingredients till the water boils. Apply the liquid on the affected part.

46. 治愈灰指甲
46. Ringworm of the Nails

(1) 用碘酒涂擦。先将患甲剥掉，然后用碘酒涂擦，每天3~5次。一个月后，有白皮的指甲慢慢变成红色，指甲也慢慢长好了。

(1) Peel off the affected nail first, embrocate the fingers with iodine tincture 3-5 times a day. One month later, the nail with white skin will become red gradually, the nail will grow slowly.

(2) 用老陈醋（要质量好一点的）半瓶，大蒜约半斤，捣碎(用刀背把它敲烂)，放在老陈醋里浸泡(无需加热)，最好是广口瓶，患者的手可以放入为佳，具体根据自己需要选择分量以及器皿。每晚将患灰指甲的手或脚放入装有大蒜的陈醋中浸泡约十五分钟，半个月基本可见效果。待新指甲慢慢长出，即可渐渐替代灰指甲，数月之后即可痊愈。

治愈原理：陈醋具有软化指甲兼杀菌作用，佐以大蒜，使得杀菌效果加倍。

(2) Half a bottle of Mature Vinegar (the quality should be good), 250g garlic, smash the garlic, then soak the smashed

garlic into the mature vinegar (without heating), put the finger of Ringworm of the Nails into the Mature Vinegar mixed with smashed garlic for 15 minutes, do it every evening, the effect will come half a month, the new nail will replace grey nails several months later.

Theory: Mature Vinegar has the functions of softening the nail and sterilization, the sterilization effect will be better if the Mature Vinegar is with garlic.

47. 天冷暖身奇方
47. Magic Therapy for Warming Body in Cold Weather

功能与原理：刺激神阙穴（肚脐），调动人体功能，舒筋活血，让血液流速加快，增加人体热量，从而达到暖身的目的。

Function and Theory: stimulate the shenque acupoint (navel), relax the muscle and speed up blood circulation, increase the body heat, thus warming the body.

适用范围：14岁以上男女均可，对年老者效果稍差。
Applicable to: people aged above 14.

配方：花椒 1g、胡椒 4g、医用橡皮胶布一小块。
Ingredients: 1g pepper, 4g piper nigrum (black pepper), a small medical sticking plastic
Preparation:

制作：
Preparation:

1. 将花椒、胡椒研末，密封备用；
1. Grind the pepper and piper nigrum into the powder, put the powder into the sealed container.

2. 把药末撒在胶布（麝香虎骨膏更好）上，即可使用。

2. Spread the powder on the medical sticking plastic (musk tiger bone plaster is recommended). The dosage gets ready for use.

使用方法：
Use Instructions:

将神阙穴（肚脐）周围洗干净，贴上胶布即可。贴一次7天左右有效。
Clean the area around shenque acupoint (navel), paste sticking plastic on the shenque acupoint, the effect will last 7 days.

48. 消除牙龈红肿
48. Removing Red and Swollen Gums

先将双手洗净，用右手中指按摩左侧的牙龈，用左手中指按摩右侧的牙龈，力度逐渐加大，时间约两分钟左右。按摩之后，立即用甲硝唑药液漱口，时间为一分钟。
Clean the hands first, then use the middle finger of right hand to massage the left gingival, use the middle finger of left hand to massage the right gingival, increase the force gradually in massaging, massage the gingival about two minutes, then rinse your mouth with metronidazole liquid

for one minute. Do it once in the morning and evening respectively.

药液配制的方法是：一片甲硝唑用 400 毫升左右的凉开水溶解。 另外，这种按摩方法还能有效地缓解牙龈萎缩。每天早晚各一次。
Method of Preparing the Liquid: Put one piece of metronidazole into 400ml cooled boiled water. Besides, such massaging can effectively alleviate the gingival atrophy.

49. 治前列腺炎
49. Prostatitis

(1) 每天晚上上床后和第二天早晨起床前，用食指和中指按在阴茎根两侧来回按摩，一手累了可换另一手继续进行。每次按摩 30 分钟，每次来回按摩约 4~6 秒钟，按摩压力以自我感觉良好为宜。坚持按摩 3 个月，病情会明显好转。
(1) After going to bed, put the index finger and middle finger on the two sides of the root of penis and massage back and forth, each massaging lasts about 30 minutes, the back and forth massaging lasts about 4-6 seconds, the massaging pressure shall be subject to good feeling. Do such massaging for three month, the obvious effect will come.

(2) 取向日葵盘（干）3 克，用凉水洗净放入杯中，水开沏泡，随喝随沏。饮此水当天见效，尿频、尿急、尿不尽、尿痛症状消失；3 天后夜尿清澈不浑浊；连饮 5 天，就可治愈前列腺炎。

(2) Take 3g sunflower head (dried), clean it with cooled water, put it into the cup, pour the boiling water into the cup, drink the water after a moment, make it again after drinking up. Drinking such water can effectively remove the symptoms of frequent micturition, urgency of urination, endless urination; the night urination is clear three days later. Drinking such water for consecutive 5 days, the disease can be cured.

50. 水土不服
50. Non-Acclimatization

到了陌生地，第一道菜应先吃水磨制的豆腐，在一定程度上可以预防和克服水土不服。豆腐对胃肠的刺激小、易吸收，能够使肠胃慢慢适应当地的饮食，老少皆宜，是克服水土不服的理想饮食。

Arriving at a new place, eat the soft beancurd first, which can prevent and overcome the non--acclimatization to some extent as the soft beancurd is little irritative to the intestines and stomach and is easy to be digested. ,

51. 治口腔溃疡
51. Oral Ulcer

(1) 常吃葡萄对治疗和防止口腔溃疡十分有效。每日吃数次，量不限，一般 2~3 天可痊愈。

(1) Eating grape is very effective in preventing and treating the Oral Ulcer, Eating the grape several times a day, the disease can be cured 2-3 days later.

(2) 用勺子舀一点纯净蜂蜜，直接涂抹在患处，让蜂蜜在口中保留一会儿，然后用白开水漱口咽下，一天两三次。一般3日内疼痛消失，溃疡面缩小，3~5日愈合。
(2) Take a spoon of honey, directly apply the honey on the affected part, keep the honey in the mouth for a moment, then drink the cooled boiled water and swallow the honey, do it two or three times a day. The pain will be removed within 3 days and the disease will be cured within 3~5 days.

蜂蜜水有利于口腔黏膜上皮细胞的修复，促进溃疡面愈合。
The homey can help the repairing of the cell on oral mucosa and promote the cure of ulcerative surface.

52. 治胃反酸
52. Stomach Acid Reflux

每次饭前吃上几口芝麻，坚持5~6天就可治好胃反酸。

Eat some sesame before having a meal, keep on doing it for five to six days, the stomach acid reflux can be cured.

53. 治扭伤
53. Sprain

根据扭伤部位的大小，取葱白200克至300克，用刀切碎之后再捣烂，放在锅中炒热到50℃左右的时候，取出敷在患处，并用医用纱布盖好。每天操作一次，七天为一个疗程，一般二至三个疗程就可治愈扭伤。
Take 200g to 300g fistular onion stalk in accordance with

the size of sprain, cut the fistular onion stalk into pieces, then mash the piece into pulp, fry the pulp in the pot till the temperature rises to 50℃, take the pulp out of the pot, apply it on the affected part and cover the pulp with gauze, do it once every day, two or three treatment courses are needed, one treatment course is seven days.

54. 治老年斑
54. Senile Plaque

每天早上空腹喝一碗醋加蜂蜜水。
Mix a bowl of vinegar and honey water, drink it every morning with empty stomach.

方法：先用凉白开水将一汤勺醋加一汤勺蜂蜜搅匀再加些热水，最少喝一小碗，多了不限。坚持半年见效。
Method: add a spoon of vinegar and a spoon of honey to a bowl, pour cool boiled water to the bowl, stir the liquids evenly, then add some hot water to the liquid, then drink a bowl of the liquid, do it for half a year, the effect will come.

55. 除鸡眼
55. Removing Helosis

先将脚放在热水里泡 15~20 分钟，然后用剪刀将鸡眼周围的坏死白皮剪掉，再用带浆的葱皮擦鸡眼口周围，最后将葱内膜贴到鸡眼口上。为防止葱掉下来，可用橡皮膏将其固定住。隔一天重复一次。
Soak the foot in the hot water for 15-20 minutes, then cut

off the Necrotized white skin around the Helosis, then use the onion skin with pulp to wipe the areas around the Helosis mouth, finally paste the endometrium of the onion on the Helosis mouth. Do it every other day.

56. 治心脑血管病
56. Cardia-Cerebrovascular Disease

将上好的黑豆洗净，凉干，用好醋泡一个星期后即可以吃。早、中、晚空腹吃，每次15粒。长年坚持必有好处，延年益寿。

Clean some good quality black soybeans and dry them, then soak the dried soybeans into good quality vinegar for one week, eat 15 such black soybeans with empty stomach in the morning, noon and evening respectively, insist on doing it around the year, the effect will come, prolonging the life.

57. 治失眠（包括高血压失眠者）
57. Insomnia (Including hypertensive insomnia)

（1）　此方主要治疗高血压失眠。醋10毫升，加一杯水中，睡前饮服，每日一次。用于治疗高血压之失眠者，饮后片刻即可入睡。

(1) Take 10ml vinegar, put the vinegar into a cup of water, drink the water before going to bed, do it once every day. You will fall asleep a moment later after drinking the water.

（2）　核桃仁、黑芝麻、桑叶各50克。捣烂如泥，做成丸，每丸3克。每次服9克，每日2次。适用于失眠较久的人。

(2) 50g walnut kernel, 50g black sesame, 50g mulberry leaf, mash these ingredients into the mud like, make the mud-like ingredients into pills, the weight of each pill is 3g, take 9g of pills orally each time, do it twice a day, this recipe is applicable to long-period insomnia.

(3) 用花生叶煎水晚上喝，三日除根。
(3) Boil the peanut leaf in water till boiled, drink the water at night, the insomnia will be removed three days later.

58. 治喑哑
58. Oligophrenia Mutism

用搪瓷容器盛上半斤食醋，里面加上三个生鸡蛋，然后煮10~15分钟，鸡蛋煮熟并保持沸腾。接着去除蛋壳，再煮10~15分钟，最后把鸡蛋连同食醋一起服下。
Pour 250g vinegar into enamel vessel, put three raw eggs into the vinegar, boil the vinegar for 10-15 minutes till the eggs are fully cooked, keep on vinegar boiling, peel off the shell of the eggs quickly, then put the eggs into the vinegar again, boil the eggs for another 10-15 minutes, then eat the egg and vinegar together.

59. 治耳鸣
59. Tinnitus

每天搓耳朵至少3次，只要有时间就搓。先搓耳廓前部，就是靠脸近的地方9下，从上而下，然后是耳廓后部，也是9下，从上而下。搓完耳朵后，再用食指堵住耳朵孔三两秒钟，然后松开。

Rub the ear with hand three times a day at least, and do it whenever possible. Rub the front part of the auricular (the area close to the face) 9 times from up to down, then rub the back part of auricular 9 times from up to down. After that, use index finger to block the ear hole for 2 or 3 seconds, then remove.

60. 治尿频
60. Frequent Micturition

(1) 摩擦肾俞穴（即腰眼）可治尿频，且疗效甚佳。
方法：晚上临睡前，坐在床上，双脚下垂，宽衣解带，舌抵上腭，调匀呼吸，收腹提肛，两手对搓发热后，紧按腰眼，用力上下搓120次，次数越多越好。

(1) Rub shenshu point (namely lumbar eye), the effect is quite good.
Method: before going to bed, sit on the bed, droop two fee, rise the tongue to push against the palate, regulate the breaching evenly, tighten up the belly, lifting the anus, rub the hands to produce heat, tightly press the lumbar eye, then rub up and down for 120 times, the more times, the effect will be better.

(2) 将淘洗干净的大米100克煮成粥，然后加入切段韭菜60克，熟油、精盐同煮，熟后温热服用，每日2~3次，有温补肾阳、固精之功效，可治疗肾阳虚、遗尿和尿频。

(2) Take 100g rice, wash it, then cook the rice into porridge, add 60g cut garlic chives to the porridge, then put pour some cooked oil and fine salt, boil them together till fully

cooked, take the dosage orally 2-3 times a day while it is warm, the recipe can improve the kidney yang and secure the essence and can cure deficiency of kidney yang, enuresis and frequent urination.

61. 治痢疾
61. Dysentery

大葱两根，去掉干皮和须根，生吃一根，第二天再吃一根，痢疾即可治愈。

Two pieces of scallion, peel off dried bark and fibrous root, eat one piece in the first day, eat one piece again next day, the Dysentery can be cured.

62. 治静脉曲张 (适用于合并浅静脉炎)
62. Varicosity (Applicable to the combined superficial phlebitis)

静脉曲张在合并浅静脉炎的情况下，每天坚持早晚用大黄泡脚 20 分钟，半月即可有明显效果。而完全静脉曲张，尤其是症状比较严重的时候，只使用大黄效果不佳。

Have a foot soak in rheum officinale liquid for 20 minutes every day, the obvious effect will come.

63. 治牛皮癣
63. Psoriasis

(1) 把大蒜放些盐捣烂如泥，敷在患处，用纱布盖好并用胶布固定，每天换新蒜泥一次。一段时间后牛皮癣便可以消除，患处只留下一块深色的斑印。
(1) Mix salt and garlic, mash them into the mud like, apply the mud-like dosage on the affected part, cover it with gauze, change the mud-like dosage once a day, the Psoriasis will be removed a period later, a deep-colored print will be left.

(2) 用自己的尿洗 7 天即愈。
(2) Wash Psoriasis with your own urine for seven days.

(3) 用刀砍榆树流出的水连抹七天。
(3) Cut the elm, the water will from the elm, collect the water and apply the water on the Psoriasis for consecutive 7 days.

64. 治瘊子
64. Wart

脸上长出一颗小米大的瘊子,后渐渐长到绿豆那么大,将蒜瓣切成小块,用以擦抹患处,先是瘊子表面出现干痂,最后竟至完全脱落,患处光洁如初,未留任何痕迹。
Cut the garlic clove into small pieces, apply the pieces on the affected part, Wart will fall off completely, no mark will be left.

65. 治轻度烫伤
65. Mildly Scalded

取鲜大蒜捣浆。用时先将患处用大蒜汁液擦拭，后用蒜泥敷。较重者第一天可换药 2~3 次，以后每天 1 次，共治疗 5~7 天。此方治疗轻度烫伤，疗效明显。

Take some fresh garlic, mash it into pulp, wipe the affected part with garlic juice, then apply the garlic pulp on the affected part. If the condition is severe, do it two to three times a day, and do it once a day later, the treatment will last 5 -7 days in total, the effect is obvious.

66. 治瘙痒
66. Pruritus

取大枣 20 枚、绿豆 100 克、猪油一匙、冰糖适量，加水共煮至绿豆开花即可服用，每天服一剂，分次服下，一般服药 3 天即可减轻瘙痒感，10 天内痊愈。

Take 20 Jujubes, 100g green bean, a spoon of lard, some rock candy, mix these ingredients and boil them in water till the green bean blooms, take one dosage a every day, the Pruritus will be alleviated three days later and will be fully cured 10 days later.

67. 治眩晕症
67. Vertigo

独活 30 克，鸡蛋（最好是红皮的鸡蛋）6 个，用水同煮。待鸡蛋煮熟时，把鸡蛋取出，把壳敲碎，再放入药锅（最好是铝锅）煮 15 分钟，去汤、去渣、吃鸡蛋，一次吃两个，每天一次，每付吃三天。轻者一付即愈，重者吃三付。

30g angelica pubescens, 6 eggs (the egg with red shell is recommended), boil them in water. When the eggs are fully cooked, take out the eggs, break the shell of the eggs, put them into the pan (aluminium pot is recommended) and boil the eggs for 15 minutes, remove the soup and residues, peel off the shell of the eggs, eat two eggs once a day, do it 3 days, the Vertigo will be cured.

68. 治哮喘
68. Asthma

(1) 杏仁半两、蜂蜜一两，水煎服治，无哮喘。
(1) Take 15g almond, 30g honey, boil them in water, drink the soup, the Asthma will be cured.

(2) 用春天起蒜时的嫩蒜 60~90 头洗干净，用蜂蜜浸泡封好后保存 6 个月。等到秋冬时打开食用，每天吃一头。坚持服用一段时间后，病情会缓解或好转。
(2) Collect 60-90 tender garlic bulbs in spring, soak them in honey and seal for 6 months, open the seal in Autumn and winter, eat one garlic bulb every day, the Asthma will be alleviated gradually.

69. 治高血压眩晕
69. Hypertensive Megrim

蜂蜜 10 克，温开水化开冲服，每日 1~2 次，长期服用更佳。
10g honey, put it into warm boiled water, drink the honey water 1-2 times a day, insist on doing it for a long time.

70. 治手脚外伤（治血）

70. Hand and Foot Injuries (Blood Disorder)

桂圆若干，食肉后将壳、核晒干，入锅炒成炭，捣碎后筛之，将其粉灰装入瓶内备用。一旦家人出现手脚外伤，敷之有奇效，愈后无痕迹。

Take Some longan, eat up the pulp, dry the shell and kernel, cook them in the pot till they become charred, mash them into pieces and screen the pieces, put the screened powder into bottle for use. Once Hand and Foot Injuries occur, apply the powder on the injuries, the effect is very good, no mark is left.

71. 治便秘
71. Constipation

(1) 每天早饭前服用几颗（块）洗净的核桃仁，或闲时随嚼，也可用豆浆一类滋补饮料冲服，能治久治不愈的便秘顽疾。

(1) Eat several cleaned walnut kernels each day before breakfast, or chew some walnut kernel at any time, or eat the walnut kernels with soybean milk.

(2) 用大米、小米各 2~3 两，加红薯 4~7 两，熬成红薯稀饭，晚饭前后食用，翌日早上，大便即可缓解，收效之速，胜过医药，且可常食，无副作用。吃一段时间的红薯，便秘可以消失。

(2) Take 60 - 90g rice and millet, 120 - 210g sweet potato, add some water in the pot, cook the ingredients into sweet potato porridge, eat the porridge before and after supper, the effect is fast and better than taking drugs. Insist on doing it for a period, the Constipation will be removed,

72. 治脑血拴脑梗塞
72. Cerebral Thrombosis, Cerebral Infarction

黑木耳10克，瘦肉150克，（猪牛羊肉均可），生姜三片，大枣5个，以上三味用六小碗水，放砂锅中煮，待煮20分钟后加入少许食盐，不要再加其它调料。每日服一次吃肉喝汤。一般患者服用4~5天即愈。
Take 10g black fungus, 150g lean meat (pork, beef or mutton is acceptable), three pieces of fresh ginger, 5 jujubes, put the ingredients into a earthen pot, add six bowls of water into the pot, boil the ingredients for 20 minutes, add some salt to the soup. Eat the meat and drink the soup once a day, the disease will be cured 4-5 days later.

73. 治骨刺
73. Spur

取50克红花浸泡在500克米醋中，一周后便可用来涂擦患部，使其软化、消除。如果严重者，多制作几次使用，效果更佳。
Take 50g carthamus tinctorius, soak it in 500g rice vinegar for one week. Apply the liquid on the affected part to soften and remove the spur. Do it several times, the effect will be better.

74. 治鼻窦炎
74. Nasosinusitis

仰头，用棉签蘸取蜂蜜，顺着鼻孔滴进去，可多滴几滴，然后用手指轻轻按揉鼻子两侧。过一会儿，鼻子就通气了。每天可滴两三次，四五天即可痊愈。

Raise head up, dip cotton swab into honey, drop the honey into the nostril, massage two sides of the nose, the nose will ventilate a moment later. Do it two or three times a day, the Nasosinusitis will be removed four or five days later.

75. 治早搏
75. Premature Beat

取黄芪15克放入杯中，加入热开水200至300毫升浸泡，随泡随服用，反复冲泡至水淡为止，每日一剂，连服五日为一个疗程。如能坚持服用一至二个疗程，常能收到消除早搏的效果。黄芪具有益气、固表、强心的功效。

Put 15g astragalus into a cup, add 200~300ml hot boiled water into the cup, soak the astragalus for a moment, then drink the water, add the hot boiled water to the cup again, till the astragalus in water becomes tasteless, take one dosage every day, insist on two treatment courses, one treatment course is five days. The astragalus has the functions of benefiting qi, securing the exterior and pumping heart.

76. 治前列腺肥大
76. Prostatic Hyperplasia

将芥末面用米醋调成糊状，摊在塑料纸上，成为比碗口大些的圆形。一小袋芥末面，可分四次用。然后把殿部尾闾（尾骨端）上部擦拭干净，再将摊好芥末面糊在尾闾往上的部位上。每日换一次即可。

Mix mustard powder with rice vinegar, stir them into starch like, then spread the starch on the plastic paper and make it into a circular biscuit with a diameter of a bowl, clean the upper part of tailbone, apply the paste-like mustard powder on the upper part of tailbone, change the starch-like mustard powder once a day.

77. 治脚裂口
77. Foot Stomium

用40℃左右的温水洗脚，泡10分钟左右，然后擦干，用温水调好芥末，浆糊状，不要太稀，用手抹在患处，穿上袜子，以保清洁。第二天再用温水洗脚，再抹，2~3次即愈。

Wash the feet with 40℃ water, soak the feet in water for 10 minutes, then wipe dry the feet, put the mustard into warm water, then stir the mustard into the starch like, apply the starch on the affected part and wear the sock to keep clean. Wash the feet in warm water, do it again, the Foot Stomium will be cured 2 or 3 days later.

78. 治跌打损伤
78. Traumatic Injury

韭菜半斤，洗净切碎捣成韭菜膏敷在患处。一般连敷三次就能痊愈。

250g Chinese chives, clean them and mash them into chive

cream, apply the cream on the affected part, do it three times, the Traumatic Injury will be fully cured.

79. 治十二指肠溃疡
79. Duodenal Ulcer

(1) 取新鲜卷心菜适量，洗净后绞取汁 200 毫升，炖温后，饭前饮服，每日 2 次，一般连服 7 天即有明显效果。

(1) Take some fresh cabbage, clean the cabbage, extract 200ml juice from it, stew the juice in the pot to warm, drink the juice before meal, do it twice a day, the obvious effect will come seven days later.

(2) 鸡蛋壳粉 90 克，陈皮 30 克。将鸡蛋壳洗净微炒，陈皮微炒，共研成细粉，每次服 3 克，每日 3 次。
(2) Take 90g eggshell powder, 30g dried orange peel, clean the eggshell, cook the eggshell and dried orange peel slightly, then grind them into fine powder, take 3g such powder orally, do it three times a day.

80. 治尿失禁
80. Urinary Incontinence

葵花根须适量，洗净，加水煎、熬至半小碗时，倒出加红糖半小勺。温服，每日 1 剂，可治疗尿失禁。
Take some sunflower root fibril, clean it, boil it in water of half a bow till boiled, pour the water into a cup, add half a spoon of brown sugar into the cup, drink the water once a

day.

81. 治骨质增生
81. Hyperostosis

(1) 用老陈醋搽揉患处，不仅有消炎止痛的效果，还能起到软化骨刺的作用。对人体新生的骨刺同样有软化的作用，且不会使老骨头受到影响。如果将一块干净的纱布用陈醋浸湿敷于患处，再用热水袋给局部加温20~30分钟，效果更好。在用老陈醋治疗的同时，不宜与其它中药混合使用，因大多数中药都含有生物碱。

(1) Rub the affected part with aged vinegar, which will alleviate the inflammation and pain and soften the bone spur, including the new bone spur, and the aged bone will not be affected. Soak a clean gauze in mature vinegar, put the wet gauze on the affected part, use the hot-water bag to heat the affected part for 20~30 minutes, the effect will be better. Do not mix other TCM drugs in this treatment.

(2) 鲨甲60克，杜仲90克，牛膝90克，鲨甲焙干研面包成12包，每日1包，日服两次，杜仲牛膝用盐水炒后，煎水分24次，送服甲面。

(2) Take 60g shark carapace, 90g Eucommia ulmoides Oliver, 90g root of bidentate achyranthes, dry the shark carapace, grind it into shark carapace powder, divided the powder into 12 bags, fry Eucommia ulmoides Oliver and root of bidentate achyranthes with salt water, then boil them in water till boiled, take half a bag of shark carapace powder orally with the boiled water of Eucommia ulmoides Oliver and root of bidentate achyranthes, take it twice a day.

82. 降血压
82. Decreasing Blood Pressure

(1) 每天吃 10 粒老醋花生，对高血压和冠心病有一定的辅助疗效。
做法：将花生仁煮熟冷却后，放在有盖的玻璃器皿中，用优质食醋浸泡 8~10 天，就可以做成老醋花生。

(1) Eat 10 Peanuts Pickled in Aged Vinegar, which has some effect on hypertension and coronary heart disease
Method: Cook the peanut kernels thoroughly, put the cooled peanut kernels into glass vessel with cover, pour good quality vinegar into the glass vessel, soak the peanut kernels in vinegar for 8-10 days.

(2) 配方：取新鲜莲藕 2.5 斤切碎，生芝麻 1 斤压碎，加冰糖 1 斤压碎。
放锅内蒸熟。取出等晾时分 5 等份。每天服用一份，一般 5 天可以降到 正常血压。较重者再服 5 天。安全可靠。

(2) Preparation: Take 1250g fresh lotus root, cut it into pieces, take 500g uncooked sesame and 500g rock candy, crush the uncooked sesame and rock candy respectively.
Put these ingredients into the pot and steam them thoroughly, then take these ingredients out and divide them into 5 equal units, take one unit orally a day, the blood pressure will decrease five days later. This recipe is safe and reliable.

(3) 取鲜芦荟叶 400~500 克，切碎，加入低度白酒 1500 克，蜂蜜 500 克，枸杞 25 克，泡上两个星期饮用，每天早晚各饮一小杯，坚持一段时间，血压便会下降。
(3) Take 400-500g fresh aloes leaf, cut it into pieces, put the aloes leaf piece into a vessel with a cover, add 1500g low-alcohol liquor, 500g honey, 25g Lycium barbarum into the vessel, cover the vessel and leave it for two weeks. Then drink one cup of the liquid in the morning and evening respectively, insist on doing so for a period, the blood pressure will decrease.

83. 肛门痒
83. Peritus Ani

芦荟有消炎杀菌的功效。早晚洗净肛门后，取一小段鲜芦荟，削去两边的刺，从中剖开，用带汁的部分擦肛门及周围，连用三天就不痒了。
Aloe has the function of sterilization and disinfection. Remove the thorns, cut the aloe into half, use the aloe juice to clean the anus and periphery, do it three days.

84. 治感冒发烧引起的咽喉发炎，红肿疼痛
84. Throat Inflammation, sore red swollen throat caused by Cold and Fever

取鲜芦荟1片（以种植一年以上者最佳），去外皮，把茎肉切成细粒，放入碗中，加入冰糖或蜂蜜。然后，放入微波炉中加热2分钟，取出连汤带渣一并食用。重症者可连续服用2~3天。
Take one piece of fresh aloe (over one year old is preferred), remove the outer skin, cut the stem into granules, put them into a bowl, add rock candy or honey into the bowl, then

heat them in microwave oven for 2 minutes, then drink the soup with aloe, insist on doing it for 2 to 3 days.

对于平时脾胃虚弱、食少便稀之人及孕妇忌用。
This recipe is not applicable to the patients of spleen-stomach deficiency and pregnant women.

85. 瘙痒症
85. Pruritus

具体方法：取芦荟叶（新叶老叶均可），切一段约3~4厘米长短，然后剖成两瓣，用叶内流出粘液的一面擦患处，可立刻止痒。
Method: take some aloes leaf (old or fresh is acceptable), cut one section with a length of 3-4cm, then dissect the section into two halves, use the juice of aloes leaf to wipe the affected part, the Pruritus will stop immediately.

86. 治贫血
86. Anemia

取绿豆和红枣各 50 克，加水 2000 毫升，放火上煮。待绿豆熬成泥状时，加红糖服用。每天一剂，15 天为一个疗程。持续服用 2~3 个疗程有疗效。
50 green bean, 50g red jujube, put them into a pot, add 2000ml water to the pot, cook them till the green bean becomes porridge like, add some brown sugar, eat the porridge every day, lasting one treatment course, a treatment course is 15 days, insist on 2-3 treatment courses, the effect will come.

87. 治溃疡性结肠炎
87. Ulcerative Colitis

鲜马齿苋 30~60 克煎水 1 碗，冲入捣烂大蒜泥 10~15 克，过滤得汁，酌加糠，1 日 2 次。
Take 30-60g purslane, put it in a pot, add a bowl of water in the pot, boil the purslane till the water boils, pour 10-15g mashed garlic to the pot, filter the soup, get the juice, add some bran to the juice, drink the juice twice a day.

88. 治胃下垂
88. Gastroptosis

配方： 良姜、均姜、陈皮(即 橙皮)、饴糖
Ingredients: falangal, dried ginger, orange peel and maltose.

上药每味各半斤（市斤），先将前三味加水煎取浓汁，去渣，再加饴糖溶化。每服一小碗，每日服三次。
Take 250g of the above ingredients respectively, boil the first three ingredients in water till boiled, take the thick juice and remove the residue, add maltose to the thick juice, drink a small bowl of the thick juice three times a day.

89. 治红白痢疾
89. Red and White Dysentery

芝麻 120 克，绿豆 120 克，两药捣碎冲服，1 日 3－5

次，即愈。

120g sesame, 120g green bean, mash the ingredients into pieces, boil them in water till the ingredients are cooked thoroughly, take the dosage 3-5 times a day, the disease will be cured immediately.

90. 治糖尿病
90. Diabetes

菜葫芦一个分7份，每份加1钱白矾，每日熬1份，3个葫芦熬21天即愈，不加盐。

Take 3 food gourds, divide one food gourd into 7 equal units, add 3g alum to each unit, boil one unit in water every day, drink the gourd soup every day, the Diabetes will be cured 21 days later.

91、治食道炎、喉哑
91. Esophagitis, Throat Dumb

烧过的煤球2个，放盒盆内捣碎，抓入2两白糖加水，放火上熬20分钟，早晚喝，三日即愈。

2 burnt briquettes, mash them in the pot, add 60g white sugar and water into the pot, boil the pot for 20 minutes, drink the soup in the morning and evening, do it for three days, the disease will be cured three days later.

92. 肺炎
92. Pneumonia

鱼腥草一把，炖荷包鸡蛋，食数口可愈。

Take a bundle of herba houttuyniae and some poached eggs, cook them in the pot till the water boils, eat the eggs, the Pneumonia will be cured a few days later.

93. 治风湿
93. Rheumatism

霜后丝瓜藤500－1000克，焙干研面，每日3次，1次2－3克，红糖水冲服。
Take 500-1000g post-frost towel gourd stem, dry it, then grind it into powder, put 2-3g such powder into the boiling brown sugar water, drink the water three times a day.

94. 腰疼
94. Low Back Pain

韭菜半斤，熬水加醋喝，不加油盐，3－5天即愈。
Take 250g garlic chives, boil it in water till boiled, then add some vinegar to the water, drink the soup, the Low Back Pain will be cured 3 to 5 days later.

95. 头晕头疼
95. Dizziness, Headache

苍耳子半两，加红糖1两，煎水喝，7天即愈。
15g fructus xanthii, 30g brown sugar, cook them in water till boiled, drink the water, the dizziness, headache will be removed 7 days later.

96. 心口疼
96. Epigastric Pain

八角茴香烧灰，乌头二钱熬水一茶杯送下，立即止痛。

Burn some star anise into ash, 6g monkshood, boil them in water till boiled, drink a cup of the water, the Epigastric Pain will be removed right away.

97. 满肚疼
97. Stomachache

用小米一把，焙干研面和水拌吃。
Take some millet, dry it and grind it into powder, mix the powder with boiled water, eat the powder mixed with water.

98. 肝炎
98. Hepatitis

用猪苦胆内的水熬开喝下，一次痊愈。
Extract the water in the gallbladder, boil the water till boiled, drink the water.

99. 妇女不孕症
99. Female Infertility

当归六钱、白芍七钱、川芎三钱、红花二钱、桃仁四钱、泽兰四钱、杞子一两。穿山甲四钱，生地八钱，香附四钱，水煎服，月经干净后每天一剂，连服三剂。

18g angelica sinensis, 21g white peony root, 9g rhizoma chuanxiong, 6g Carthamus tinctorius, 12g peach seed, 12g Herba Lycopi, 30g Wolfberry, 12g pangolin scales, 24g Rehmannia root, 12g rhizoma cyperi, boil these ingredients in water till boils, take one dosage orally every day after menstrual bleeding stops, and take three dosages consecutively.

100. 闭经
100　Amenorrhoea

益母草一两，煎药一碗加黄酒服下即愈。

30g herba leonuri, boil it in water till boils, drink the soup with yellow rice wine.

101. 月经不调
101　Irregular Menstruation

月季花十朵，煎水加红糖，酒引连服半月愈。

Take 10 Flos Rosae Chinensis, boil them in water till boils, add some brown sugar to the water, take the soup orally after drinking a little wine, do it for half a month.

102. 经疼
102. Menstrual Pain

棉籽一把，新瓦焙干碾粉服三钱立即止疼。（特效）
Take a handful of cotton seeds, dry them on new tile, grind the dried cotton seeds into powder, take 9g such powder orally, the Menstrual Pain will be removed right away.

103. 白带
103. Leucorrhea

白果十五个，炖江米稀饭食，每天一次，七天痊愈。
Take 15 semen ginkgoes, stew glutinous rice in water into porridge, eat the semen ginkgo with porridge, do it for seven days, Leucorrhea will be removed.

104. 下奶奇法
104. Magic Method for Promoting Lactation

黑皂角籽七个，生的，研沫开水送下，一小时自下。
Take seven raw seeds of black Gleditsia sinensis Lam, grind the seeds into powder, take the powder orally with boiled water, the effect will come one hour later.

105. 经血不止
105. Persistent Menstruation

莲蓬壳烧灰，热酒服下，日服二次，每次二钱,，七天即愈。
Burn lotus receptacle into ash, take 6g such ash orally twice a day with hot wine, Persistent Menstruation will be removed seven days later.

106. 大便出血
106. Gastrorrhagia

豆腐渣二斤，炒黄拌白糖吃，立止。
100g soybean curb residues, fry and stir the soybean curb residues till they become yellow, eat the soybean curb residues with white sugar, Gastrorrhagia will stop right away.

107. 阳痿病
107. Impotence

阳起石、枸杞子三钱，加红糖水煎服，效果奇佳。
9g actinolite, 9g fructus lycii, boil them in the brown sugar water till the water boils, drink the soup, the effect is very good.

108. 小儿夜哭
108. Baby Night Cry

五倍子三钱。
用法：炒后研成细沫，将药面涂在小儿肚脐周围。即可治小儿夜哭安然睡眠。
9g gallnut, fry the gallnut and grind it into foam, apply the foam on the periphery of navel of the baby, the baby will fall asleep quickly.

109. 百虫入耳
109. Verminal Invasion Ear

猫尿滴耳百虫自出。（大蒜咬断抹猫鼻子猫自尿）
Drop the cat urine into ear, the bugs will come out. (cut off the garlic, apply the garlic on the nose of the cat, the cat will urinate).

110. 治脚干裂
110. Foot Crack

食盐二斤，加水六斤，烧开煮化稍冷洗脚，七天即愈。

Take 1000g salt, put the salt in the water of 3000g, cook the water till boils. Wait a moment, wash feet in the water, do it for seven days, the Foot Crack will be cured.

111. 脚鸡眼、刺猴
111. Toe Corns and wart

用大麻子1粒，捣烂抹上用胶布贴上，一次即愈。
One hempseed, mash the hempseed, apply the mashed hempseed on the affect part, cover it with gauze. Toe Corns and wart will be cured once for all.

112. 治烧（烫）伤
112. Burn Injury (Scald)

羊屎蛋7个放火上焙丁研面，杏油调和涂伤处，日涂三次，并能止疼而又不留伤疤，三日即愈。
Take 7 Sheep feces balls, dry them on fire, grind them into powder, mix the powder with sesame oil, apply the powder on the injury three times a day, the dosage can kill the pain and leaves no scar, do it for three days.

113. 毒蛇咬伤
113. Venomous Snake Bite

烟袋油擦伤口，再用清水将烟袋油冲下来喝，如觉香甜，即伤重应多喝，如果觉苦，即伤轻，应少喝。
Apply tobacco pipe oil on the wound, wash down the tobacco pipe oil with clear water, drink the tobacco pipe oil, if the patient feels it is fragrant and sweet, it means the wound is serious, drink it more; if the patient feels it is bitter, it means the wound is light, drink it less.

114. 遗尿、下淋
114. Enuresis, Trickling

用五年以上的葵花杆瓢子二尺，水煎一碗喝下，一次即愈。
Take 2/3 meter of sunflower stem pulp aged above 5, cut into several sections, boil them in water till the water boils, drink the water, the disease will be removed once for all.

115. 蛲虫病
115. Enterobiasis

用烟袋油抹肛门，虫自死，永不复发。
Apply the tobacco pipe oil on the anus, the bugs will be killed, the Enterobiasis will never happen again.

116. 治通身水肿
116. Edema

用红瓤西瓜一个，麦糠埋住，把糠用火点着，等火灭后吃西瓜，每天吃一个，3－5天痊愈。
Take a watermelon with red pulp, bury it in wheat bran, fire the wheat bran. After the fire extinguishes, eat the watermelon, eat one such watermelon every day, the Edema will be cured 3 to 5 days later.

117. 小便不通
117. Urinary Stoppage

高粱杆上皮，越老越好，熬水喝，不加盐，两日即愈。

Take some sorghum stalk skin (the older one is preferred), boil it in water till the water boils, drink the water, do it for two days, the Edema will be cured.

118. 大便结症
118. Stool Indigestion

菠菜一斤，猪油（大油）1两，放锅内炒吃，三日痊愈。

500g spinach, 30g lard, fry them in the pot, and eat them,

the Stool Indigestion will be fully cured three days later.

119. 身上痒
119. Body Itch

用荆芥熬水洗患处，两次除根。
Boil the Schizonepeta tenuifolia in water till the water boils, wash the affected part with the water, do it twice, the Body Itch will be removed completely.

120. 尿床
120. Bed-Wetting

鸡肠子四服，洗净用新瓦焙干研沫开水冲服，日服两次，每次二钱，七天即愈。
Four chicken intestines, clean them with water, dry them on the new tile, grind the dried chicken intestines into powder, put the powder into boiling water, drink 6g of such water each time, and drink it twice a day, the Bed-Wetting will be fully cured seven days later.

121. 耳炎
121. Otitis

蛇皮一节，香油泡一天用油滴耳即愈。
A section of snake skin, soak the snake skin in sesame oil one day, drop the sesame oil into the ear, the Otitis will be cured right away.

122. 常见眼疾
122. Common Eye Diseases

黑豆二两、白菊花七钱，煮沸熏眼，效果良佳。
60g black soybean, 21g feverfew, boil them in water till water boils, then fumigate the eyes, the effect is good.

123. 搭背疮
123. Sore on the Back

用秦艽三钱，天花粉二钱，研面牛乳调抹，即好。
9g gentiana macrophylla, 6g Snakegourd root, grind them into powder, mix cow milk with the powder, eat it, Sore on the Back will be cured right away.

124. 睡觉多梦
124. Dreaminess after Sleeping

当归、生地、红花、牛膝各三钱，积壳、赤芍、甘草各二钱，桔梗、川芎各一钱半，桃仁四钱煎服。二剂可安然睡眠而梦少。
Take 9g angelica sinensis, 9g dried rhizome of rehmannia, 9g flos carthami and 9g Achyranthes bidentata, 6g fructus aurantii, 6 Red Peony Root and 6g liquorice, 4.5g radix platycodonis and 4.5g rhizoma chuanxiong, 12g peach kernel, mix and boil them in water till the water boils, drink the soup orally, do it twice.

125. 鱼骨卡喉自化

125. Fishbone Stuck in Throat

轻者慢喝陈醋一两，鱼骨即软可吞下；
Drink 30g mature vinegar, the fishbone will soften, swallow the fishbone.

126. 瘫痪
126. Paralysis

槐枝、桃枝、柳枝、椿枝、茄枝，共切碎合煎水三桶。用大盆浸洗。如冷加热立洗。后睡床盖被让出汗避风，洗数次即愈。

Take some sophora japonica branch, peach juvenile branch, willow branch, toon branch, eggplant branch, cut them into pieces, boil the pieces of them in three barrels, pour the hot boiled water in a big basin, soak the feet in the big basin for a moment till the water cools, then go to sleep, cover the body with quilt, making the body sweat, avoid the wind, do it several times, the effect will come.

127. 面下粉刺
127. Acne

蔓菁子研沫。加入雪花膏，每天晚上涂抹，数日即愈。

Grind turnip seed into powder, add vanishing cream to the powder, apply the mixed on the face every evening, do it several days, Acne will be removed.

128. 刁斜风（口歪眼斜）
128. Deviation of Mouth and Eye

将蓖麻籽研烂，左歪涂左，右歪涂右，复正即速去之。

Grind castor seed into pulp, apply the pulp on the deviated side, and remove the pulp after the deviation returns to normal.

129. 疝气
129. Hernia

人中白二钱，红糖一两。共研细末，黄酒送下，日服二次，早晚各一次。半月即愈。

6g Depositum Urinae Hominis, 30g brown sugar, grind them into powder, take the powder orally with yellow rice wine twice a day, do it in the morning and evening respectively, the Hernia will be cured half a month later.

130. 白癜风
130. Vitiligo

用青核桃皮焙干研沫，小磨香油调和，每日抹三次，半月除根。

Take some walnut green husk, grind them into powder, mix the powder with ground sesame seed oil, stir the mixed, apply the mixed dosage on the affected part, do it for half a month, Hernia will be removed half a month.

131. 紫癜风
131. Lichen Planus

硫磺 3 分，密陀僧 3 分，共研细面，用醋调，贴患处。

Take 0.09g sulphur, 0.09g lithargite, grind them into powder, mix the powder with vinegar, apply the mixed dosage on the affected part.

132. 晕车
132. Carsickness

食醋 1 两，开水 2 两，拌匀上车前喝下，可立止。
30g vinegar, 60g boiled water, mix them and stir the liquid evenly, drink the liquid before getting aboard

133. 解煤气中毒
133. Gas Poisoning

用浓茶，好醋各一碗混合，分三次服用，每次间隔半小时，一个半小时后，彻底痊愈。
Take a bow of strong tea and a bowl of quality vinegar, mix them, drink the mixed liquid every half an hour, do it three times, the Gas Poisoning will be removed completely.

134. 立止鼻血
134. Stop Nosebleed

用头发烧成灰，吸入鼻孔，可立止，男用母发，女用父发。
Burn the hair into ash, inhale the ash into nostril, the nosebleed will stop right away. If the patient is male, use the hair of his mother; if the patient is female, use the hair of her father.

135. 立止刀伤出血
135. Stop Bleeding Knife Wound

鸡毛灰涂患处,立止流血,并不感染。
Apply chicken feather ash on the affected part, the bleeding will stop at once without infection.

136. 绣球风
136. Skin Diseases of the Scrota

苦参 20 克,地肤子 15 克,水煎,外洗,每日二次。
20g sophora flavescens, 15g fructus kochiae, boil them in water, wash the affected part with the liquid, do it twice a day.

137. 食物中毒
137. Food Poisoning

绿豆一大把,生甘草三钱。加水煎几次服下。
Take a handful of green bean, 9g fresh licorice, boil them in water till the water boils, drink the water for several times.

138. 肥胖症
138. Obesity

硫苦 5 克，红糖 20 克为一服，冲服 7 天，特效。
5g magnesium sulfate, 20g brown sugar, mix them in the pot, pour the boiling water into the pot, drink the water for seven days, the effect is very good.

139. 夜盲眼
139. Night Blindness

白水煎羊肝，羊肝煮熟吃，不加盐料。
Boil the Sheep Liver in clear water till the Sheep Liver is cooked thoroughly, then eat the Sheep Liver.

140. 预防麻疹
140. Measle Prevention

西河柳（河边柳叶）、芫荽各 50 克。水煎洗全身。
Take 50g Cacumen Tamaricis (riverside salix leaf), 50g Coriandrum sativum, boil them in water till water boils, then wash the body with the water.

141. 扁平疣
141. Flat Wart

牛唾液，涂患处。
Apply cow salivary on the affected part.

142. 积滞
142. Indigestion

鸡内金1个，黑丑5克。焙干研成细沫，每日1次，开水送服。

Take 1 Endothelium Corneum Gigeriae Galli, 5g semen pharbitidis, dry and grind them into powder, take the powder orally with boiled water, do it once every day.

143. 狐臭
143. Body Odor

古矾10克，硫磺5克，苦参6克，蛇皮5克。用上药研成细沫，生姜片蘸上药涂患处，每日2次。

Take 10g dried alum, 5g sulphur, 6g sophora flavescens, 5g snake skin, grind them into powder, dip the ginger slice into the powder, then apply the ginger slice on the affected part, do it twice a day.

144. 治痢疾
144. Dysentery

每日每次用冷开水冲服40毫升蜂蜜，最好在饭前1小时或饭后2~3小时服用，成人每日3次，小儿用量酌减，婴儿用量控制在30克，混合在稀粥、牛奶或豆浆中喂服。

Pour cooled boiled water into 40ml honey, drink the honey water 1 hour prior to meal or 2-3 hours later after meal. An adult shall drink the homey water three times a day. For a child, mix 30g honey water with thin porridge, milk or soybean milk, then eat the thin porridge or drink the milk or soybean milk.

145. 治低色素性贫血、头晕失眠
145. Hypochromic Anemia, Dizziness Insomnia

每天早晚用鸡蛋1个，开水冲熟后，加入蜂蜜30克服用（最好用深色蜜，置瓷盅内隔水蒸8~10分钟备用）
Open an egg, put it into a pot, pour boiling water into the pot. After the egg is well-cooked, add 30g honey (the dark honey is recommended, steam the dark honey in a pot for 8-10 minutes) to the egg, eat one such egg in the morning and evening respectively.

146. 治咽干口燥、手足心热
146. Dry throat and mouth, feverishness in palms and soles

大梨一个挖孔，蜂蜜50克放入其中，蒸熟食之，一日2个连服数日即可。
Take a big pear, dig a hole in the pear, then pour 50g honey into the hole, steam the pear till it is well cooked, eat two such pears a day, do it for several days, the effect will come.

147. 口臭
147. Ozostomia

白蔻仁适量。每次取一粒，放口中含嚼，每日 3 次。
Take appropriate quantity of the seeds of Amomum cardamomum, put one seed into the mouth and chew the seed, do it for three times a day.

(The End)

www.ingramcontent.com/pod-product-compliance
Lightning Source LLC
Chambersburg PA
CBHW060411190526
45169CB00002B/858